PRIMARY CARE TRAINING AND DEVELOPMENT

The Tool Kit

Lynn Talbot

and

Denise Pora

Foreword by

Rosey Foster

Radcliffe Medical Press

Radcliffe Medical Press Ltd
18 Marcham Road
Abingdon
Oxon OX14 1AA
United Kingdom

www.radcliffe-oxford.com
The Radcliffe Medical Press electronic catalogue and online
ordering facility.
Direct sales to anywhere in the world.

British Library Cataloguing in Publication Data

A catalogue record for this book is available from the British Library.

ISBN 1 85775 909 5

Typeset by Aarontype Limited, Easton, Bristol
Printed and bound by TJ International Ltd, Padstow, Cornwall

CONTENTS

FOREWORD

Primary care is at the forefront of the NHS. The evolution of general practice into primary care and the management of first-line patient services and care continues to be a challenge for those who work within it and those who are part of the NHS infrastructure to support it.

At the time of writing, the details of the new GMS Contract have yet to be finalised. Primary care groups are still coping with the transition into primary care trusts (in England). The NHS in Scotland, Wales and Northern Ireland progresses via devolution at a different pace, using different organisational structures and language. Nevertheless, primary care managers throughout the UK will benefit by taking protected time to read and reflect on the contents of this tool kit as it provides a fresh approach to training and development.

Management within primary care will be based, in the future, on evidence of competence. One approach for understanding what will be required and how to begin is contained in the text. The tool kit is aimed at all those who have, or wish to have, an active role in developing primary care management. As new management models emerge across organisational boundaries, this role may well be the general practice manager who is retained by the primary care organisation (PCO) to develop new training strategies for local practices in collaboration with PCO staff. There are a number of GPs who assume a management role and this tool kit with its competence profile is therefore a good starting point for understanding future requirements and when recruiting a new practice manager.

The authors have structured the tool kit in seven sections, each with an explanatory text for developing policies, strategies and procedures, with useful checklists and activities which act as a prompt for further discussion. Particularly helpful are the sections on mentoring and the introduction of a critical incident diary – new learning tools for managers to develop their reflective practice in keeping with other healthcare colleagues.

The time taken to work through the eight key competence areas following all the guidance will put managers in a prime position to implement the next stages of the NHS Plan and the outcome of the GMS Contract negotiations.

Rosey Foster FIHM
Deputy Chief Executive
Institute of Healthcare Management
January 2003

ABOUT THE AUTHORS

Lynn Talbot is a Director in McLaren Parry working as a change consultant, in particular around the modernisation agenda, redesigning services to meet the needs of today's world, and specialising in facilitating teams, project management and management skills training.

Denise Pora combines working in an acute NHS Trust as a senior human resources advisor with her role as an independent consultant, specialising in personal, management and organisational development. She is a Fellow of the Chartered Institute of Personnel and Development.

INTRODUCTION TO THE TOOL KIT

The NHS is changing at a relentless pace and nowhere more so than in primary care. Clinical, management and administrative roles in general practice have developed significantly over the past ten years resulting in many new challenges and demands on individuals and teams.

One consequence of this is that a planned approach to the training and development of the whole primary care team has become more important than ever to support the introduction of new services and ways of working and primary care managers now need both strong general management and development skills.

This tool kit is a practical, flexible resource for individual and team training and development in primary care. It provides a step-by-step guide to identifying, planning and implementing training and development and includes a competence profile developed with primary care managers to provide a framework for developing abilities and behaviours, underpinning knowledge and skills needed now and in the future.

Section 1

USING THE TOOL KIT

PURPOSE

This section describes how managers and others working in primary care can use the tool kit.

THE TOOL KIT

The tool kit can be used by:

- new and experienced practice managers to plan their own training and development and that of their team(s) and practice(s)
- other professionals working in general practice and primary care trusts who have responsibilities for supporting the development of practice management
- clinical and administrative staff who want to develop a career in practice management.

It provides a step-by-step guide to:

- identifying current and future roles
- assessing individual and team strengths and development needs
- planning training and development and choosing development methods
- successfully implementing individual, team and organisational development plans.

Each section gives detailed suggestions about activities to undertake and easy-to-use tools. All the tools can be photocopied and adapted to suit individual needs.

You can work sequentially through the tool kit at your own pace, or use the resources in different sections as the need arises, as in the following examples.

- Managers who want to review their development needs and establish a plan to manage their career will find it helpful to work through the pack sequentially.
- The competence profile is a good starting point for anyone who is recruiting a new practice manager and needs to develop a job description and person specification.
- Primary care trust (PCT) development managers can use the competence profile to plan the curriculum for training events for primary care managers.
- Anyone facing the challenge of implementing major changes for the first time and who needs some support will get ideas from the sections on planning and implementing development.
- Line managers and those being appraised will find the sections on assessing needs, planning and implementing development plans useful when preparing for annual performance reviews.

FORMAT OF THE TOOL KIT

Sections 3 to 7 provide guidelines for individuals working on their own *personal development* and tools and suggestions for *line managers* and *trainers* who may be supporting individual members of staff, teams or organisational training and development. Each section is divided into two parts – the first gives advice and suggested activities and the second provides training and development tools.

Section 2

TRAINING AND DEVELOPMENT POLICIES, STRATEGIES AND PROCEDURES

PURPOSE

This section explains the purpose of organisational and team training and development policies, strategies and procedures. It gives guidelines and tools to help decide what is needed and how to develop and implement them.

PURPOSE OF TRAINING POLICIES, STRATEGIES AND PROCEDURES

By developing training and development policies, strategies and procedures you can make sure you:

- know what you are trying to achieve now and in the future by developing explicit links between training and development and organisational or team goals
- plan and use your resources effectively and enable rational and productive prioritisation of training and development that supports team/organisational goals (*see* Section 5)

- communicate with everyone in the team or organisation and establish a common expectation and understanding in the team or organisation about:
  - what is to be done and why
  - who is entitled to what and why
  - who is responsible for what and when

- identify the need for change and take action through a regular, systematic review of progress.

DEFINITIONS

TRAINING AND DEVELOPMENT POLICY

Describes the team or organisation's approach to training and development – it must be consistent with the strategy.

The policy should be reviewed annually.

TRAINING AND DEVELOPMENT STRATEGY

Describes what is to be achieved through training and development in support of the organisation or team's future vision (which is often described through business strategies, plans and long-term objectives).

Usually long term – three to five years – but can be less in a fast-changing environment.

TRAINING AND DEVELOPMENT PROCEDURE

Describes how the organisation administers and manages training and development in order to apply its policy and successfully implement its strategy.

Procedures can take on a life of their own and it is vital that they are reviewed annually to ensure they are still providing a mechanism for meeting the team or organisation's needs.

LINKING POLICY, STRATEGY AND PROCEDURE

The links between a policy and a strategy should be obvious, as should the ways in which the procedure supports them both.

For example:

Practice objective
- To extend the range of health promotion services available for patients over the next three years.

Relevant part of the training and development policy
- The commitment of the practice to encourage and support the professional development of staff to achieve its goals.

Supporting element of the training and development strategy
- To improve and develop the health promotion skills of practice nurses over the next three years.

Key area of the training and development procedure
- The identification of training needs through the annual objective setting and appraisal process – making the connection between the practice's objective and the individual's appropriateness and wish to develop his/her health promotion skills.

DEVELOPING POLICIES, STRATEGIES AND PROCEDURES

TRAINING AND DEVELOPMENT POLICIES

Every organisation has a training and development policy – that is the way it makes sure its workforce has the skills it needs to perform its function success-fully. The policy may not be written down, but it will exist. At one extreme an organisation may always seek to recruit fully trained and qualified staff for all of its functions and provide only essential induction training. The policy of this organisation is that it accesses a competent workforce by buying it.

Unwritten policies will often determine who has access to training and development – funding and time off for training is available to one group of staff, but not for another. The reason may be historical, or even economic (one group of staff is easier to recruit if individuals leave because of a lack of development or career progression). Nothing is written down, but everyone knows this is the team or organisation's policy.

By deciding to develop and publish your policy you are making a public statement about the role of training and development in your team or organisation.

It is important that you fully think through the implication of your policy. For example, if you say your team or organisation encourages the career and personal development of individuals, does this include support (financial or through giving paid, or unpaid, time off work) of activities that will not result in direct benefits for the organisation?

Some organisations support all forms of personal development or growth for their employees and may provide funding for them to learn new skills that will never be applied at work (e.g. handicrafts or sports). Others encourage career development and support learning that may lead to an employee gaining a promotion and moving to another part of the NHS.

Your policy needs to consider practical issues, such as the resources available, and it may be necessary to give priority to some areas or groups – for example, health and safety training, or mandatory annual training for clinical staff.

The guiding principle is to ensure your policy meets the needs of your team or organisation, and is a concise statement of what you actually intend to do – it should not raise expectations that you cannot (or do not plan to) meet. If your aspirations of what you would like to do are greater than what you can deliver in practice, *always* stick to what you can deliver.

Manager's/trainer's activity 1

Developing a team or organisational training and development policy

1 Your decision to develop a policy already demonstrates that you think training and development has a key role to play in the future success of your team or organisation. Using the examples and checklist in Section 2 tools (*see* pp 15–16), draft a policy statement for your team or organisation. You might do this on your own, or with a colleague or group of colleagues.

2 As with a strategy, it is important that all key stakeholders fully understand and endorse a training and development policy. Identify the key stakeholders who need to endorse the policy, and how and when you will present it to them and seek their views.

3 Make sure everyone in the team or organisation knows about and understands the policy by, for example:

- circulating a copy of the policy (either a paper copy or via e-mail)
- putting copies on notice boards and/or websites
- discussing it at team meetings
- including details in regular newsletters
- organising special short briefing sessions to explain the policy and answer any questions.

Review your policy once a year and ask the following questions.

- Does this represent what we are doing in practice?
- Is this what we should be doing – do we need to change anything?

TRAINING AND DEVELOPMENT STRATEGIES

A training and development strategy details what you plan to achieve through training and development to support your team or organisation's future medium- to long-term vision. Before starting you need to know what that vision is, or if there is one.

Manager's/trainer's activity 2

Identifying the need for a team or organisational training and development strategy

The first step in developing a team or organisational training and development strategy is to review existing plans, strategies or goals and the external environment.

You may be developing your training and development strategy as part of an overall team or organisational planning process, or where there are clear and agreed plans and objectives for the team or organisation. If you are, go on to *manager's/trainer's activity 3* (*see* p 11).

You might find various plans and objectives that are not comprehensive or even complementary, or there is a general intention that everything should stay much the same as it is now, with necessary changes being introduced in an ad hoc way (which is extremely unlikely to be a successful strategy in today's world).

In these circumstances there are three options.

1 Bring together all the plans, strategies and objectives you can find, including those that are only available verbally, e.g. in someone's head. You may need to pull together a number of documents, or spend time talking to a range of people to get a comprehensive picture of where the team or organisation is going. Confirm they represent the team or organisation's objectives with the key stakeholders and ensure any conflicting priorities or plans are addressed. You should also consider what is happening outside your team or organisation, in the NHS or wider world – what are the implications of these changes? (*See* Section 2 tools.) Go on to *manager's/trainer's activity 3* (*see* p 11).

---

2 Work with your team or key colleagues in the organisation to develop a shared vision of where the team or practice is going and what you want to achieve in the next three years. Identify and address any gaps or inconsistencies in any existing objectives or plans. Remember to consider changes outside your team/organisation. Go on to *manager's/trainer's activity 3 (see* p 11).

The Section 2 tools are designed to help you develop a training and development strategy in support of team or organisational goals, but some can usefully be adapted or applied to the development of team or organisational objectives/goals.

Both of the above options potentially represent a significant investment of time, effort and skill. The pay-off of a shared vision of the team or organisation's future, which gives a sound foundation from which strategy can be developed to achieve the vision, is likely to justify your investment.

If the first two options are not appropriate:

3 Abandon the idea of developing a comprehensive team or organisational strategy and identify whether or not there are any current significant needs or changes (i.e. not comprehensive but still substantial team/organisational plans for the future). For example:

- new services for patients, e.g. a walk-in centre
- new systems, e.g. a new computer system, patient-held records
- new roles e.g. healthcare assistants, specialist nurse practitioners
- a new National Service Framework (NSF).

If you identify one or more significant changes or needs, move on to *manager's/ trainer's activity 3 (see* p 11).

In the absence of any clear team or organisational goals for the future or significant change(s) planned, there is little point in attempting to develop a training and development strategy.

A training policy and supporting procedures will be supportive of maintaining the ongoing objectives of the team/organisation.

Teams and organisations often fail to develop robust training and development strategies even when they have good medium- to long-term objectives. Sometimes this is because it all looks 'too difficult' or, ironically, because everything appears straightforward. In both cases the result can be the failure to fulfil an achievable vision, missed opportunities, the alienation of staff or the expenditure of much more time and effort than was necessary.

A training and development strategy does not have to be a long document – a page or two may be enough – and developing a strategy need not be a complex or laborious task. However, it is essential to go through all the steps – even if the answers appear obvious. More often than not the process flags up issues that would have been missed entirely, or would have only come to light when they become a problem.

Manager's/trainer's activity 3

Developing a team or organisational training and development strategy

1 Review your team/organisation's future objectives, strategies and/or plans and changes in the external environment. Identify the possible workforce implications. (*See* Section 2 tools.)
2 Review your team/organisation's current staffing and identify likely or possible changes over the period of time you are addressing. (*See* Section 2 tools.)
3 Compare the two analyses you have carried out on the workforce implications of your future objectives and your current and future staffing. Identify the overall staffing implications for the team/organisation. (*See* Section 2 tools.)
4 Consider your options for addressing the possible workforce implications and select the one(s) most likely to succeed in achieving the team/organisation's future objectives. This should include assessing the resource implications of each option. (*See* Section 2 tools.) The training and development options selected become your training and development strategy from which you will be able to develop annual team/organisational training and development plans and clarify what your policy needs to be.
5 Ensure the strategy is fully understood, accepted and endorsed by *all* those who have a role in implementing it (e.g. supplying resources, releasing staff for training and those who are to undergo training and development).

An example of objectives translated into a training and development strategy

Organisational vision
- Reduce doctors' workloads over the next two years by introducing general minor illness clinics led by a specialist nurse practitioner.

Training and development strategy
- **Objective:** Develop and run an in-house national vocational qualification (NVQ) training programme for healthcare assistants to support existing practice nurses. (Resource implications over next two years: programme development and running costs – £X.)
- Support nurse practitioners to qualify as specialist nurse practitioners (Resource implications over next 18 months: costs of training and additional staff cover – approximately £X.)

TRAINING AND DEVELOPMENT PROCEDURES

Your procedure describes how training and development will be administered and managed in your team or organisation.

A good procedure will ensure you apply your policy and achieve your training and development strategy efficiently and fairly. The shorter and easier a procedure is to understand and apply, the more likely it is to be successful.

Manager's/trainer's activity 4

Developing a team or organisational training and development procedure
You may already have informal, unwritten rules or custom and practice that already exist, or a situation where you are starting with a blank piece of paper. In either case you will need to gain the understanding and acceptance of key stakeholders in the team/practice to what you are proposing.

1 Identify any formal/informal written/unwritten rules or custom and practice that already exist.
2 Using the *checklist for developing a training and development procedure* in Section 2 tools (*see* p 16), write a draft procedure.
3 Note any areas where you are suggesting a change from what currently happens and ask yourself why. You will need to have a clear (and reasonable) explanation if asked about the change by someone who prefers the existing approach.
4 Consult with the key stakeholders who need to endorse the procedure.
5 Make sure that everyone in the team/organisation knows about and understands the procedure. Study point 3 of *manager's/trainer's activity 1* (*see* p 8) for suggested ways of communicating the policy.

Section 2
THE TOOLS

EXAMPLE TRAINING AND DEVELOPMENT POLICY STATEMENT

XYZ Practice recognises that training and development are fundamental to its continuing efficiency and success and is committed to working in partnership with all staff to support activities that contribute to the achievement of the practice's goals.

To help achieve this objective and at the same time fulfil its duty to staff, the practice will develop its human resources by a systematic approach to its training and development requirements.

It is the policy of the practice to support and encourage all staff to develop to the full extent of their ability or personal choice. All managers must ensure staff have access to opportunities for training and development which are in line with the needs of the practice. Individual members of staff are responsible for working with their line manager to identify and meet their own needs to achieve and maintain a satisfactory level of performance in their job.

Funding and paid time off to support training and development will be given at the discretion of the line manager and budget holder.

Notes

This brief statement makes the following clear.

- The practice makes a direct link between training and development and the achievement of objectives – i.e. its purpose. In this organisation training and development activities are not undertaken simply because they are 'a good thing to do', nor are they a 'reward' for good behaviour. Any activities that cannot show a clear link to the needs of the practice are likely to be refused.
- Training and development is available for all staff.
- Training and development will be planned and managed systematically.
- Both individuals and their managers have responsibilities.

CHECKLIST FOR DEVELOPING A TRAINING AND DEVELOPMENT PROCEDURE

1 How will individual, team and organisational training and development needs be identified (e.g. through the annual business plan, through team objectives and plans, through individual appraisal processes)?

2 Who is responsible (e.g. Practice Manager responsible for identifying organisational needs from the practice business plan, managers/supervisors responsible for ensuring appraisal happens)?

3 How are training and development activities authorised and recorded (e.g. individuals complete a form, which is signed by their manager)?

4 Is it necessary to confirm what are considered to be training and development activities that are covered by the procedure – courses, workshops, open-learning courses, seminars, visiting another organisation, shadowing someone for a day, meeting with a mentor?

5 Are any records of training and development kept centrally, or do managers or members of staff hold everything? Central record keeping helps with monitoring and evaluation, but could be time consuming.

6 What are the guidelines for managers for deciding if and how much funding and time off to give for training and development? Guidelines might include:

- the training was agreed as part of a personal development plan
- there are clear, specific and agreed outcomes expected from the training
- it represents good value for money
- undertaking it will not have an adverse impact on the individual's ability to perform his/her role, or on the workload of others in the team/organisation.

Specific guidance may be helpful on:

- payment of fees for examinations, professional subscriptions and course set books, e-learning
- travel expenses
- time off for examinations and revision, visits to mentors, open-learning studies, e-learning.

7 How will training and development be monitored and evaluated?

8 What happens if there is a disagreement?

- Is the manager's decision final?
- Who has the final say?

DEVELOPING A TRAINING AND DEVELOPMENT STRATEGY: ANALYSING EXTERNAL FACTORS

PEST ANALYSIS

A PEST analysis can be used to identify external factors that may have an impact on the team or organisation. Under each of the four headings **P**olitical, **E**conomic, **S**ocial, **T**echnological, consider changes that will or may happen during the period you are planning for and how they could affect you.

For example:	
Political • Government plans for the NHS. • Government legislation – e.g. employment law, health and safety.	**Social** • Patient expectations of primary care. • Demographics – e.g increasingly elderly population.
Economic • State of the national economy e.g. impact on health, labour markets. • Developments in private healthcare sector.	**Technological** • New developments, e.g. medical technology, pharmaceuticals • Pace of technological change, e.g. internet – more informed patients.

Assessing the workforce implications of team or organisational plans

Purpose

This exercise provides you with a step-by-step guide to assessing the workforce implications of team and organisational objectives in terms of their impact on the numbers of staff and roles needed, the skills and knowledge needed and consequences for working patterns.

It will give you a comprehensive overview of the expected workforce requirements, including their impact on your current workforce.

It will be most effective and useful when carried out with the people responsible for developing and implementing the objectives as the process may identify new issues. As a minimum you must test your analysis with them.

Step 1
Review each part of the vision/all objectives and ask the question:

What is the likely impact of achieving the vision/objectives or implementing the change on:

1   **Staff numbers and roles – will we need:**

- More staff? If yes:
  - Which roles?
    - Existing roles?
    - New roles?
    - Some new/some existing?
    - Are there options using different mixes of roles?*
  - How many more?
  - By when?
  - All at once or over a period of time?
    - What is the timescale?

---

* Using staff with different 'skill mixes', e.g. healthcare assistants working in support of practice nurses undertaking tasks such as blood pressure monitoring and venepuncture.

- Less staff? If yes:
  - Which roles?
  - How many less?
  - By when?
  - All at once or over a period of time?
    - What period of time?
- Same number of staff? If yes:
  - Which roles?
    - Existing roles?
    - New roles?

2   Skills and knowledge – will staff need new skills?

- What skills?
- Who will need them?
- When?

3   Working patterns – will it be necessary for staff to:

- Work different shift patterns?
  - What are they?
- Work in different locations?
  - Where?

STEP 2
ANALYSE THE ANSWERS TO STEP 1 FOR ALL PARTS OF THE VISION/OBJECTIVES AND IDENTIFY THE OVERALL WORKFORCE IMPLICATIONS IN TERMS OF:

1   Impact on staff numbers and roles

- How many more of a particular existing role?
  - When will they be needed?
- How many less of a particular existing role?
  - When will they no longer be needed?
- How many of any new roles?
  - When will they be needed?

2 Impact on skills and knowledge

- What new skills and knowledge will be needed?
  - By whom?
  - When?

3 Impact on working patterns

- What will be different?
  - For whom?
  - From when?

ASSESSING THE CURRENT WORKFORCE

1 Collect the following information about each member of staff.

Name								
Current role								
Location (if appropriate)								
Pattern of work and hours								
Age/length of time before retirement								
Qualifications: • achieved • studying for								
Skills								
Previous roles/experience								
Future career plans								

2 Collate the information for the whole team/organisation and identify the following:

Current workforce	
• Total number of staff in each role (e.g. Patient Focused Services, Prescribing, Practice Management and Administration)	
• Total number of hours available weekly in each role	
• Pattern of hours available in each role	
• Location of staff in each role	
• Expertise available – qualifications, skills and experience not currently used	
Future developments – current workforce	
• Roles becoming vacant due to retirements (what and when)	
• New qualifications and skills becoming available (what and when)	
• Other expected developments (e.g. a part-time member of staff may indicate he or she plans to seek full-time work within the next six months)	

ASSESSING THE CURRENT WORKFORCE: AN EXAMPLE

1 Collect the following information about each member of staff.

Name	Caroline Henderson
Current role	Practice receptionist
Location (if appropriate)	Vinery Road Health Centre
Pattern of work and hours	Monday to Thursday 8.30 am to 12.00 pm, Friday 2.00 pm to 3.30 pm (15.5 hours a week)
Age/length of time before retirement if less than five years	DOB 22.9.73/retirement +5 years away!
Qualifications: • achieved • studying for	RSA Diploma for Personal Assistants, RSA II Word Processing None
Skills	Reception, general administration
Previous roles/experience	Secretarial and financial administration
Future career plans	Has shown interest in taking on more practice administration/management work. Particularly interested in IT and computers.

2 Collate the information for the whole team/organisation and identify the following.

Current workforce	
• Total numbers of staff in each role (e.g. Patient Focused Services, Prescribing, Practice Management and Administration)	**Practice Management and Administration:** Five staff (3 × receptionists, 1 × general business administration/finance, 1 × Practice Manager)
• Total number of hours available weekly in each role	**Practice Management and Administration:** 120 hours weekly (45 hours reception, 37.5 hours general business administration/finance, 37.5 hours practice management)
• Pattern of hours available in each role	**Practice Management and Administration:** Vinery Road: Reception – Monday to Thursday 8.30 am to 12.00 pm and 2.00 pm to 3.30 pm. Vinery Road: Business administration/finance and practice management – Monday to Friday 8.30 am to 5.00 pm. Charles Street: Reception – Monday and Wednesday 8.30 am to 1.30 pm, Friday 8.00 am to 1.30 pm
• Location of staff in each role	**Practice Management and Administration:** Vinery Road – Receptionists: Caroline and Brigit / Admin/finance: Sam / Practice management: Sylvia. Charles Street – Receptionist: Joyce
• Expertise available – qualifications/skills/experience not currently used	**Practice Management and Administration:** Sam: Certificate in Management. Caroline: finance – administration and monitoring

Future developments – current workforce	
• Roles becoming vacant due to retirements (what and when)	**Practice Management and Administration:** Practice Manager: Sylvia retiring next July
• New qualifications and skills becoming available (what and when)	**Practice Management and Administration:** Brigit due to complete Practice Manager Development Programme in February
• Other expected developments (e.g. a part-time member of staff may indicate he or she plans to seek full-time work within the next six months)	**Practice Management and Administration:** Caroline wants to increase her hours when Ben starts secondary school next September

FUTURE WORKFORCE NEEDS

Month/year	*Planned change/development*	*Workforce needs/implications:* • *additional roles (new or existing)* • *roles becoming redundant*
For example:		
June 2004	• Completion of extension at Vinery Road and new General Minor Illness Clinic starts	• Additional new role: specialist nurse practitioner
July 2004	• Closure of Charles Street surgery on expiry of lease • Practice Manager retires	• Charles Street receptionist role becomes redundant • Replacement needed – by end May to allow handover?
September 2004	• Vinery Road receptionist (Caroline) wants full-time hours now son at secondary school	• Up to an additional 22 hours available in practice administration at Vinery Road

CHECKLIST FOR ASSESSING WORKFORCE OPTIONS

NEW ROLES OR MORE OF AN EXISTING ROLE

- Is it likely that we could recruit someone with the skills/experience needed? How soon? How much will it cost?
- Could we reallocate duties among existing staff to fill the role?
- Could one of our existing employees be promoted into the role? Does anyone have skills/qualifications we are not using? What would the implications of this be for the team/organisation?
- Would any existing employees take the role as a sideways move to enhance their future career prospects by widening their experience? What are the implications of this for the team/organisation?
- Does anyone want to increase the hours he or she works to fill the role?
- Could the role be filled by paying overtime?
- Could one of our existing employees be trained to fill the role? Is there time? How much would it cost? What would the implications be?

REDUNDANT ROLES*

- Are there any other opportunities within the team/organisation now or in the foreseeable future?
- Could the individual be trained to fill a different role in the team/organisation?
- Are there appropriate ways of creating a role, e.g. other staff reducing their working hours?

---

* These questions are intended to help identify options; they do not address employers' statutory responsibilities in the event of redundancy.

EVALUATING WORKFORCE OPTIONS

SWOT ANALYSIS

A SWOT (**S**trengths, **W**eaknesses, **O**pportunities and **T**hreats) assessment is a useful tool for considering the viability of an idea or making choices between options. Simply consider which aspects of the option(s) are strong, weak and represent opportunities or threats for the team or organisation.

For example: Sam to replace Sylvia as Practice Manager when she retires.

Strengths

- Sam has strong financial and business management skills.
- He wants the job (may look elsewhere for opportunities otherwise).
- Plenty of time for smooth handover and transition between Sylvia and Sam.

Weaknesses

- Sam is not a strong people manager – need for training; is there time?
- Not introducing 'new blood' and ideas into the practice.

Opportunities

- May be opportunities for Caroline to take on some of Sam's finance work – and offer Joyce at least some hours at Vinery Road.

Threats

- Brigit may leave when she gets her Practice Manager's qualification.
- Sam is not a strong supporter of IT – what about the new computer system?

Section 3

THE PRIMARY CARE PRACTICE MANAGEMENT COMPETENCE PROFILE

PURPOSE

This section provides a framework for identifying what primary care managers need to be able to do now and in the future.

THE COMPETENCE PROFILE

The primary care practice management competence profile is a framework covering eight key areas of performance.

These are:

- managing work
- managing change
- managing other people
- developing other people
- working with other people
- communicating
- analysing and using data
- personal effectiveness.

The profile describes the competences – abilities and behaviours underpinning knowledge and skills – needed in each of the areas. The balance and level of competences needed by individuals will vary depending on the nature and scope of their role.

Using the profile

The profile can be used to:

- clarify your role
- review performance
- identify current and future training and career development needs
- clarify the roles of those you manage, review their performance and identify their training and career development needs
- provide information for job descriptions and person specifications
- help prepare questions for selection interviews
- help prepare for appraisal meetings with your line manager or those you manage.

Personal development

Personal development activity 1

Using the competence profile to describe your current and future role

1   Use the competence profile on pages 35–38 as your framework to think about your current job. Identify which of the key areas of performance it includes. Are any more important than others?

- Put a tick against all those needed in your job now.
- Place an additional tick against any that are particularly important.

2   Think about how your job might change in the next 12 months. Will you need to do anything new as a result? Will any areas of performance become more or less important?

- Put *three ticks* against any *additional* key areas of performance you expect to need in the next year.
- Finally, put another tick against any existing areas that will become even more important in the coming months.

You might find it helpful to get other peoples' ideas about the future – your line manager or other primary care managers, for example.

Next steps for individuals
When you have clarified your role and identified possible changes in the next 12 months, go to Section 4 to assess your strengths and development needs.

LINE MANAGERS AND TRAINERS

USING THE PROFILE IN RECRUITMENT AND SELECTION

The competence profile can be used in recruitment and selection by helping to clarify and describe job roles and the skills and knowledge needed to fulfil them. The competences can also aid selection by acting as a guide to the choice and use of assessment methods.

Recruitment
The 'key areas of performance' part of the competence profile can be used when developing new job descriptions or reviewing existing ones before recruitment.

Person specifications can be derived from the 'skills' and 'knowledge' sections of the profile.

Templates for job descriptions and person specifications, and examples based on the profile, are given in Section 3 tools.

Selection
Successful selection of the best person for the job depends largely on the accuracy of your measurement of how well each candidate fulfils the criteria of your person specification.

When choosing selection methods it is important to identify which criteria you expect each method to measure. The Section 3 tools give a comprehensive breakdown of suggested selection methods for the skills and knowledge of the primary care practice management competence profile.

SHOP RECEIPT

DATE ...8-9 MAY 2003 ....

QTY	TITLE OF BOOKS	PRICE
	HEALTH BOOKS FROM	
	PRIMARY CARE EXPO	
	2 x	39-51
TOTAL PRICE		
PAYMENT METHOD		39-51

Management Law Finance Health Management Health and Safety British Standards Maps and Guide Superplan	**the Stationery Office** **68 –69 BULL STREET BIRMINGHAM B4 6AD** **Tel: 0121 236 9696 Fax: 0121 236 9699**	**TSO**

VAT NUMBER GB 676 733 690   ---   **THERE IS NO VAT ON BOOKS**

Section 3

THE TOOLS

PRIMARY CARE PRACTICE MANAGEMENT COMPETENCE PROFILE

1   Managing work

Key areas of performance

☐ Sets targets/objectives and identifies the action needed to achieve them
☐ Plans and prioritises work for self and others
☐ Identifies and implements appropriate systems to achieve practice targets/objectives
☐ Delegates tasks with appropriate authority

Skills	Knowledge
• Objective setting • Planning and prioritisation • Time management • Chairing meetings/leading group discussions • Delegation • Problem solving • Decision making	• Planning and managing rotas and appointments systems • NHS complaints procedures • Health and safety regulations • Business planning • Service specification, contract tendering and management processes

2   Managing change

Key areas of performance

☐ Identifies the need for change resulting from internal and external issues
☐ Actively seeks opportunities to improve performance
☐ Develops, implements and evaluates change plans that take account of the internal and external context

Skills	Knowledge
• Facilitation • Planning and prioritisation • Creativity	• Change management theory and techniques • Current developments in primary care, the wider NHS and external environment

3   Managing other people

Key areas of performance

☐ Acts as a role model for the behaviour that is expected within the practice
☐ Makes sure staff understand what is happening in the practice, PCT and wider environment
☐ Makes sure staff know what is expected of them and that they have the capability and capacity to deliver it
☐ Monitors and provides feedback on performance, intervening if necessary
☐ Builds an effective team and creates a co-operative and harmonious environment
☐ Identifies and addresses conflict within the team

Skills	Knowledge
• Objective setting • Delegation • Motivating others • Managing and resolving conflict • Team building • Providing constructive feedback • Interviewing: for selection, grievance and discipline	• Human resources good practice and relevant employment law for recruitment, selection, employment contracts, discipline, grievance and equal opportunities • Appraisal processes • Current developments in primary care, the wider NHS and external environment

4   Developing other people

Key areas of performance

☐ Identifies training and development needed by individuals and groups of staff
☐ Actively seeks to identify potential in others and provides opportunities for them to realise it

Skills	Knowledge
• Questioning • Active listening • Coaching • Mentoring • Providing constructive feedback	• How to identify group and individual training and development needs • Training and development methods and opportunities

---

5   Working with other people

Key areas of performance

☐ Builds effective working relationships with all staff in the practice
☐ Develops external networks to gather and share information and understanding of the wider environment
☐ Negotiates with individuals and groups internally and externally to achieve workable outcomes
☐ Gains the support and commitment of others through effective influencing
☐ Acts as an ambassador for the practice when dealing with the public and other professionals from outside the NHS
☐ Deals sensitively and effectively with emotional or aggressive patients

Skills	Knowledge
• Influencing • Networking • Negotiation • Active listening • Questioning	• Developments in primary care, the wider NHS and external environment • Local groups and networks • Techniques for dealing with aggressive patients

6   Communicating

Key areas of performance

☐ Written and verbal communications get the message across clearly and consistently
☐ Effective on a one-to-one basis and in group settings
☐ Uses questions, active listening and non-verbal communication to seek information and understanding
☐ Adopts the appropriate style for the audience

Skills	Knowledge
• Active listening • Questioning • Presentation • Report writing • Note taking • Facilitation	• Non-verbal communication

7   Analysing and using data

Key areas of performance

☐ Makes accurate calculations using financial and other numerical data
☐ Gathers, analyses and interprets financial, numerical and other data to aid the clarification of problems, identifying options and making decisions

Skills	Knowledge
• Numeracy • Problem solving • Decision making	• Financial forecasting and planning • Income and expenditure accounting • Book keeping • Personal Medical Services (PMS) and/or the Red Book • Items of Service (IOS) regulations • PAYE regulations • Local and/or statutory requirements for special pay, e.g. maternity, sick • Data protection requirements • NHS Information Management and Technology (IM and T) requirements

8   Personal effectiveness

Key areas of performance

☐ Manages own time effectively
☐ Manages own stress and controls emotions appropriately
☐ Understands own impact on others and adapts style appropriately to the situation
☐ Seeks and acts on constructive feedback from others
☐ Knows own strengths and weaknesses
☐ Open to new ideas, willing to change and adapt
☐ Actively seeks opportunities for training and personal development

Skills	Knowledge
• Time management • Stress management • Feedback • Assertiveness	• Self-awareness • Training and development methods and opportunities

JOB DESCRIPTION TEMPLATE

Job title:

Reports to:

Purpose of the job:

Principal resources controlled:

- staff
- budgets
- premises

Key tasks:

Contact with others:

Major challenges of the job:

Decision-making authority:

Signatures

Job holder .... Date ....

Line manager .... Date ....

EXAMPLE JOB DESCRIPTION BASED ON PRIMARY CARE PRACTICE MANAGEMENT COMPETENCES

Job title: Practice Business Manager

Reports to: The partners of the practice

Purpose of the job: Operational and strategic management and development of practice in line with the partners' objectives, NHS requirements and within available human and financial resources.

Principal resources controlled:

- staff
- budgets
- premises

Key tasks:

Managing work

1 Responsible for development, production and overseeing implementation of the annual practice business and training plans.
2 Develop and co-ordinate systems to achieve practice targets/objectives, working closely with the Head Receptionist and Nurse Co-ordinator.
3 Work with partners to ensure good health and safety practices are implemented and maintained, and legislative requirements met.
4 Oversee the maintenance of practice premises and equipment, ensuring contracts for cleaning and maintenance are let and managed effectively.
5 Attend and contribute to practice meetings; prepare agenda and minutes.

Managing change

1 Keep up to date with all NHS changes and developments affecting primary care locally and nationally, including regular liaison with PCT staff.
2 Work with partners to identify change resulting from internal and external issues; developing and implementing strategies and plans to introduce new services and manage changes effectively.

Managing other people

1 Issue staff contracts and maintain contracts and personnel files of all employed staff.

2   Implement effective appraisal and development systems that ensure staff know what is expected of them and that they have the capability and capacity to deliver it.
3   Work with partners to build an effective team and create a co-operative and harmonious environment, identifying and addressing conflict as necessary.
4   Ensure staff understand what is happening in the practice, PCT and wider environment.

Developing other people
1   Identify team and individual training and development needs of employed staff, and develop strategies and plans to meet them.
2   Actively seek to identify potential in others and provide opportunities for them to realise it.
3   Support the development of attached staff, and contribute to their training.

Financial and information management
1   Develop, manage and control practice budgets and financial systems.
2   Maintain financial records and prepare financial forecasts.
3   Oversee the administration of financial schemes including pensions, maternity and sick pay.
4   Oversee and develop the operation of the practice computer network.
5   Ensure compliance with NHS Information Management and Technology requirements.
6   Ensure compliance with the Data Protection Act.

Contact with others:
- Build effective working relationships with all staff in practice.
- Develop external networks to gather and share information.
- Act as an ambassador for the practice when dealing with the public and other professionals from outside the NHS.

Major challenges of the job:

Decision-making authority:

Signatures

Job holder .... **Date** ....

Line manager .... **Date** ....

PRACTICE MANAGEMENT PERSON SPECIFICATION TEMPLATE

Job title:

	Essential	Desirable
Skills		
Knowledge		
Experience		

PRACTICE MANAGEMENT PERSON SPECIFICATION EXAMPLE

Job title: Practice Business Manager

	Essential	Desirable
Skills	• Objective setting, planning and prioritisation • Delegation, problem solving, decision making • Creativity • Motivating others, managing and resolving conflict • Team building • Questioning, listening, providing constructive feedback • Influencing, negotiation, networking • Report writing • Numerical • Time management, stress management • Assertiveness	• Chairing meetings/leading group discussions • Facilitation • Coaching, mentoring • Presentation • Note taking
Knowledge	• NHS complaints procedures • Health and safety legislation • Business planning • Change management theory and techniques • Current developments in primary care • Human resources good practice and employment law • Identification of training needs and methods • Income and expenditure accounting, financial planning	• Planning and managing rotas and appointment systems • Contract tendering and management • Current developments in the wider NHS • Appraisal processes • Techniques for dealing with aggression and violence • Local NHS and primary care networks and groups • Data Protection Act 1998 • NHS IM and T developments • PMS • PAYE regulations
Experience	• Staff management • At least three years in primary care management	• Practice Manager role • Working in PMS pilot practice

PRIMARY CARE PRACTICE MANAGEMENT COMPETENCE PROFILE: SUGGESTED SELECTION METHODS

PURPOSE

It is essential that the criteria listed in your person specification are tested by your selection process. This table makes suggestions for selection methods that can be used to assess the primary care practice management competences.

---

1   Managing work

- Interview – ask candidates for examples of systems they have identified the need for and implemented (may follow up examples from application form)
- Interview – standard questions for candidates on how they would handle a patient's complaint
- In-tray exercise – candidates are asked to deal with set of tasks relevant to the job that require them to plan and prioritise work and delegate tasks

2   Managing change

- Interview – ask candidates for examples of previous change management
- Group exercise – set candidates a group task to develop plans to implement NHS change (testing approach to change management and current developments in NHS/primary care)

3   Managing other people

- References from current/previous employers
- Personality questionnaires providing insight into management style
- Interview – ask candidates for examples of managing poor performance (may follow up examples from application form)

4   Developing other people

- Case study – candidates to describe their approach to a given scenario either at interview, as part of in-tray exercise or as part of pre-prepared interview for panel
- References from current/previous employers

5	Working with other people

- Group exercise – candidates will demonstrate their ability to influence, negotiate, listen actively and question
- Personality questionnaires providing insight into relationships with others

6	Communicating

- Pre-prepared presentation to panel
- Interview – may have one-to-one and panel sessions
- In-tray exercise – test written communication
- Group exercise – will provide evidence of listening, questioning and non-verbal communication

7	Analysing and using data

- In-tray exercise requiring analysis and calculation using financial, numerical and other data
- Psychometric tests of verbal, abstract and numerical reasoning
- Interview – problem-solving questions for candidates to test ability to 'think on feet'

8	Personal effectiveness

- Group exercise – tests candidates' ability to manage stress, control emotions and adapt style appropriately
- Interview – ask for candidates' perceptions of their strengths and weaknesses, and their approach to their own development
- References – from current and previous employers

Section 4

ASSESSING STRENGTHS AND DEVELOPMENT NEEDS

PURPOSE

This section gives you tools and ideas to help assess individual and team strengths and development needs using the primary care practice management competence profile.

PERSONAL DEVELOPMENT

INDIVIDUAL SELF-ASSESSMENT

When making your own assessment of your strengths and development needs, take time to really think about your performance and challenge yourself. Identify at least one recent example to support your assessment and don't allow past mistakes to colour your view too much.

You could also keep a *critical incident diary* (*see* Section 4 tools, pp 64–65) to gather information by recording, analysing and learning from what happens during your working day. Simply keep a diary for a week or two and write down your key experiences – for example, things that went well or badly, and insights you get into your performance from your own observations and feedback from others. Review your diary at the end of the period and spot any trends or issues that suggest strengths or development needs.

Personal development activity 2

Assessing your competence

1   Assess yourself against the competence profile using the *competence assessment questionnaire* and guidance notes in Section 4 tools (*see* pp 57–63). If there were any areas of the competence profile that you decided were not relevant to your role now or in the next 12 months when you completed *personal development activity 1*, do not include them in your assessment.

2   Note your results below – what insights have you gained about your strengths and development needs? Are there any patterns?

3   Look at the competence profile in Section 3 tools (*see* pp 35–38), and review the list of underpinning skills and knowledge for each key area of performance. Write down those you think you need to develop.

Getting feedback from others

As well as assessing your competence yourself, it is best to get information from as many other perspectives as possible to get a rounded picture of your strengths and development needs. Different people will be able to provide valuable feedback depending on the aspects of your job they see you performing.

To get useful and usable feedback from other people, it is vital that you:

- are clear about the sort of feedback you want
- choose people who can and will provide useful information.

Identifying the feedback you want
Decide if there are particular areas of your performance that you are interested in learning more about – possibly areas where you think you could improve. The more specific you can be about the feedback you want, the more likely you are to get helpful information from others. It is a good idea to write down what it is you want so you are clear about what you are asking for. Remember: if you ask someone for feedback on your performance you may get some surprises – good and bad.

Choosing people who can and will provide useful information
Choosing the right person or people to give you feedback is crucial. The right person will:

- be someone whose opinion you value (if you don't value his or her opinion the feedback will be of no use to you)
- have enough knowledge of your performance overall, or in your chosen areas, to give feedback based on sound evidence
- be honest with you
- have the time and willingness to discuss the feedback with you
- be someone who has direct, recent experience of your performance.

The following people *may* be able to offer valuable information:

- your line manager
- other colleagues, e.g. in the practice, PCT or outside
- your staff
- your mentor or coach, if you have one.

Whoever you decide to ask for feedback, always ask for evidence of your performance to back up general comments. It is possible that the feedback you get from others will not be consistent, with one person rating you highly on something that another thinks is a development need for you. This may be an area that you want to discuss with one or both of them, before deciding if it is a competence you need to develop.

Remember: seeking feedback using the competence assessment questionnaire is an art, not a science.

Personal development activity 3

Getting feedback from others
1   Identify any areas of your performance you are particularly keen to get feedback on, and list them below.

2   Decide whom you are going to ask for feedback (probably between two and five people) and list their names below.

3   Ask each of them to give you feedback using the *competence assessment questionnaire* as a framework (*see* the guidance notes for using the competence assessment questionnaire in Section 4 tools, pp 57–58)

DRAWING UP YOUR LIST OF STRENGTHS AND DEVELOPMENT NEEDS

The *competence assessment questionnaire* and your *critical incident diary* should give you useful information about your strengths and development needs, but you may decide to use data you have gathered from other sources as well, for example:

- a recent appraisal discussion with your line manager or a member of staff
- feedback from a training course
- feedback from a job interview
- comments or suggestions from your mentor.

Personal development activity 4

Reviewing strengths and development needs

1   Review the information you have gathered from your own assessment and feedback from others about your strengths, development needs and the underpinning knowledge and skills you need to develop.

2   Also consider any other recent feedback or insights into your strengths and development needs (from appraisal discussions etc.).

3   Identify any common themes between the feedback you have had from others and your own views about your performance. Are there any conflicts? Note particularly if you have one or more rating of 1 or 4 in any areas of the competence assessment questionnaire.

4   Now write a list below of your strengths and your development needs, and the underpinning skills and knowledge you need to develop.

Next steps for individuals
Go to Section 5 to start planning your training and development.

LINE MANAGERS AND TRAINERS

ASSESSING OTHER PEOPLE'S NEEDS

There are a number of ways the competence profile can be used to assess the training and development needs of practice management and administration staff.

Line managers often experience extreme difficulty both in identifying the training needs of their staff and agreeing effective methods to meet them. This often results in staff attending courses and workshops that have little or no impact on their current job performance or future career prospects.

An effective process of training needs analysis need not be laborious and can result in the need for less rather than more time and money being spent on development activities, while leading to real improvements in performance. A checklist for managers assessing the training and development needs of their staff is provided in Section 4 tools (*see* pp 66–67).

Manager's/trainer's activity 5

Using the competence profile to assess someone else's needs

1   Use the *competence assessment questionnaire* in Section 4 tools and identify the areas of performance that are relevant to the member of staff's role – both currently and any you expect to develop over the next 12 months. (Adapt the questionnaire to the role if necessary – for example, if the individual does not have responsibility for managing or developing other members of staff.)

2   Consider the person's current performance in each of the key areas and rate them on the 1 to 4 scale. Always record *at least* one example of their performance in the past 12 months that provides evidence for your rating.

3   Highlight any new areas where the member of staff is not currently required to perform that will develop over the next year (i.e. where you are not able to score them).

4   Take each of the areas where you have rated performance 1 or 2 (or 3 if the area is one where the acceptable level of performance is for the job holder to demonstrate the competence very often or always) in turn, and review the relevant skills and knowledge section of the competence profile (*see* Section 3 tools). Identify the skills and/or knowledge needed to improve performance.

5   Next consider the key areas you expect to develop over the next 12 months, and use the competence profile to identify the skills and knowledge the job holder will need to develop.

6   You may also ask the job holder to complete steps 1 to 5. (Whether or not this is appropriate will depend largely on the individual's ability and motivation to contribute to the identification of the training and development needs in this way.)

7   Meet with the job holder and work through the competence assessment questionnaire (or questionnaires if you both completed the exercise). The examples of performance will help to establish a shared understanding of the required level of performance and areas for training and development.

8   Once training and development needs have been agreed, use Section 5 tools to identify the best way of meeting them. (It may be helpful to work through the *assessing needs and options* tool and *developing skills and knowledge matrices* together.)

Manager's/trainer's activity 6

Using the competence profile to identify the content of a primary care management development programme

The competence profile and assessment questionnaire can be used to identify the priority training and development needs of a number of individuals in similar roles within the same practice or across a number of practices.

To establish commonly held needs, the questionnaire should be completed by:

- all programme participants – prioritising the key areas of performance of the role using the competence profile and scoring their current performance against the questionnaire
- programme participants' line managers – prioritising the key areas of performance of the role using the competence profile and scoring their member of staff's current job performance against the questionnaire
- a selection of participants' subordinates – scoring their line manager's current performance against the questionnaire.

The purpose of the exercise is to generate a prioritised list of group needs that can then be developed into a training and development programme. There will be no feedback to individuals and all responses should be completely anonymous.

Section 4
THE TOOLS

PRIMARY CARE PRACTICE MANAGEMENT COMPETENCE ASSESSMENT QUESTIONNAIRE

Self-assessment

1   Think about your performance in each of the competency areas and rate yourself on the 1 to 4 scale. Include examples of your recent performance, as evidence to support your self-assessment will help ensure that you are being fair to yourself – for example, not allowing a mistake made five years ago to distort your view of your performance in a particular area.

2   Review your scores and identify any patterns or areas where you have particular strengths or development needs.

Asking other people to give you feedback using the questionnaire

1   Approach the people you identified in *personal development activity 3* (*see* p 50) and ask if they are able to help you. Explain what you want, why you want it and the timescale you are working to and then ask if they can help.

2   Agree a time when you can discuss the feedback they have given you. It is not recommended that you use the questionnaire to seek anonymous feedback, as you will not be able to follow up any comments or ratings you need to discuss or do not understand.

3   Give them a copy of the competence profile (*see* Section 3 tools, pp 35–38) and the questionnaire. Go through the instruction sheet on the next page with them to make sure they understand what they need to do.

Instructions for completing the questionnaire to give someone else feedback

The purpose of this questionnaire is to provide a framework to assess the way individual managers perform against the competence profile for primary care practice managers and give them information about their strengths and development needs.

The questionnaire can be used to provide feedback to others on their performance or as a self-assessment tool. The person who has asked you to complete the questionnaire for him or her will tell you how he or she is using it.

To complete the tool:

1   Think about how the person does his or her job, under each of the headings, and give a rating on the 1 to 4 scale based on your experience of him or her at work.
2   Give evidence that supports your rating in the comments/suggestions box. The best sort of evidence is examples from your recent experience – for example 'acted on the feedback given about the new rota', 'identified the need to change the appointments system'. If you do not know about the person's performance in a particular area, leave that section blank rather than guessing.
3   Use the information about underpinning knowledge and skills on the primary care practice management competence profile to suggest possible development needs.

It will probably take you 30 to 45 minutes to complete the questionnaire.

Rating scale

The scale is based on how often you think the person you are rating demonstrates the competence as described.

1 = Very rarely or never
2 = Sometimes
3 = Usually
4 = Very often or always

QUESTIONNAIRE

Managing work	1	2	3	4	Comments/suggestions
• Sets targets/objectives and identifies the action needed to achieve them					
• Plans and prioritises work for self and others					
• Identifies and implements appropriate systems to achieve practice targets/objectives					
• Delegates tasks with appropriate authority					
Managing change	1	2	3	4	Comments/suggestions
• Identifies the need for change resulting from internal and external issues					
• Actively seeks opportunities to improve performance					
• Develops, implements and evaluates change plans that take account of the internal and external context					

Managing other people	1	2	3	4	Comments/suggestions
• Acts as a role model for the behaviour that is expected within the practice					
• Makes sure staff understand what is happening in the practice, PCT and wider environment					
• Makes sure staff know what is expected of them and have the capability and capacity to deliver it					
• Monitors and provides feedback on performance, intervening if necessary					
• Builds an effective team and creates a co-operative and harmonious environment					
• Identifies and addresses conflict within the team					

Developing other people	1	2	3	4	Comments/suggestions
• Identifies training and development needed by individuals and groups of staff					
• Actively seeks to identify potential in others and provides opportunities for them to realise it					

Working with other people	1	2	3	4	Comments/suggestions
• Builds effective working relationships with all staff in the practice					
• Develops external networks to gather and share information and understanding of the wider environment					
• Negotiates with individuals and groups internally and externally to achieve workable outcomes					
• Gains the support and commitment of others through effective influencing					
• Acts as an ambassador for the practice when dealing with the public and other professionals from outside the NHS					
• Deals sensitively and effectively with emotional or aggressive patients					
Communication	1	2	3	4	Comments/suggestions
• Written and verbal communications get the message across clearly and consistently					
• Effective on a one-to-one basis and in group settings					

	1	2	3	4	Comments/suggestions
• Uses questions, active listening and non-verbal communication to seek information and understanding					
• Adopts the appropriate style for the audience					
Analysing and using data	1	2	3	4	**Comments/suggestions**
• Makes accurate calculations using financial and other numerical data					
• Gathers, analyses and interprets financial, numerical and other data to aid the clarification of problems, identifying options and making decisions					
Personal effectiveness	1	2	3	4	**Comments/suggestions**
• Manages own time effectively					
• Manages own stress and controls emotions appropriately					
• Understands own impact on others and adapts style appropriately to the situation					

	1	2	3	4	Comments/suggestions
• Seeks and acts on constructive feedback from others					
• Knows own strengths and weaknesses					
• Open to new ideas, willing to change and adapt					
• Actively seeks opportunities for training and personal development					

USING A CRITICAL INCIDENT DIARY

The purpose of keeping a critical incident diary is to identify your strengths and development needs by gathering information from everyday working experiences.

Simply keep a diary for at least a week and up to a month and write down your key experiences each day. Record things that go well or badly, and feedback you get from those you work with through their comments and observations.

If possible, fill in the 'What happened?' column as things happen during the day, and add any immediate observations about why and possible implications. At the end of each day, review what you have written on your diary sheet and write down further thoughts about why and possible implications.

At the end of the time you have set for keeping your diary, review all you have written and identify any trends or patterns that give you insights into your strengths and development needs.

You can use a copy of the diary sheet as shown opposite, or transfer the format into your personal diary or notebook depending on what will be the easiest way of keeping your critical incident diary close to hand at all times during your working day.

You may also find it helpful to discuss what you learn from keeping a diary with someone else – your line manager, a mentor or colleague.

CRITICAL INCIDENT DIARY

Date	What happened?	Why?	The possible implications are . . .

LINE MANAGER'S CHECKLIST FOR ASSESSING TRAINING AND DEVELOPMENT NEEDS

	Question	Comments/action
1	Do you have a complete and up-to-date understanding of the purpose of the job, the principal resources controlled and key tasks?	
2	Are there any areas where the job holder's performance falls below the acceptable standard?	
3	If yes, can you give more than one recent example of this?	
4	If no, is it possible you are allowing one mistake or error to colour your judgement?	
5	Do you know what knowledge, skills or experience would improve performance?	
6	If no, does the job holder's performance fall below the acceptable standard because of attitude or motivation rather than lack of skill, knowledge or experience? If yes, this is a performance management issue, not training and development.	
7	Do you expect any changes that will affect the purpose of the job, principal resources controlled or key tasks in the next 12 months?	

Question	Comments/action
8 Will any of these changes result in the need for the job holder to develop new skills, knowledge or experience?	
9 Does the job holder have career plans or aspirations?	
10 If yes, do you believe they are realistic? Are you prepared to support the job holder? What knowledge, skills and experience can you offer the job holder in the next year that will help achieve the plans?	

Section 5

PLANNING TRAINING AND DEVELOPMENT

> ## PURPOSE
>
> This section gives step-by-step guides to developing individual, team and organisational training and development plans.

PERSONAL DEVELOPMENT

WHAT IS A PERSONAL DEVELOPMENT PLAN?

A good personal development plan (PDP) is your individual map, setting out:

- how to improve your performance in your current job
- how you want your career to develop
- what you are going to do
- when you will do it
- who will help you.

Your personal development plan is a live document, which must be part of an ongoing process that helps you to:

- continue to improve in your current job
- monitor your progress
- identify and plan the training and development you will need as your job changes and your career develops.

It can be a vital tool in conversations with your line manager or other people who are helping you with your training and development, such as a coach or mentor.

DEVELOPING YOUR PDP

Now you have identified the key competences you want to develop, you can start to identify how. To successfully develop the competence, you need to identify:

- an effective way of developing the particular competence
- a training or development method that fits your personal needs, preferences and circumstances.

Personal development activity 5

Identifying priorities for the next year

1   Look at the competence profile you prioritised against your job in *personal development activity 1 (see* Section 3) and the list of development needs you drew up in *personal development activity 4 (see* Section 4).

2   Write down any of the competences that you gave two or three ticks (i.e those you think are important now or will be in future) *that also appear on your list of development needs.* These are your *priority areas for development* in the next year.

3   Write down any remaining development needs from the list you compiled during *personal development activity 4.* These are areas to address if an opportunity arises and time/resources allow in the next year or in the longer term.

Personal development activity 6

Assessing your needs and options

Use the *assessing needs and options* proforma in Section 5 tools to consider each of your priority development needs for the next year in turn (or all of your development needs if you think you will have sufficient resources to address them). This will help identify the development methods that are best for you. It is important to do this to ensure that you choose a method(s) that fits your needs and any constraints you face. The sorts of things you might think of are given in the following example.

Competence: Working with other people – developing external networks to gather and share information and understanding of the wider environment

---

1   What do I need?

To develop my networking skills and improve my knowledge of local groups and networks

---

- How much do I already know? Am I starting from scratch?
- Do I need to develop my knowledge?
- Do I understand the theory but need to practise?
- Could I practise on the job, or do I need a low-risk environment away from work?

    (a) Local practice managers group organised by PCT, have never attended it
    (b) Need to know more about networking tools and techniques and practise them

---

2   How much time do I have?

- How quickly do I need the competence? Do I need it urgently?
- Can I afford to take time away from work to develop it? How much?
- Am I prepared to spend some of my own time developing it?

    (a) Need to develop over the next 12 months
    (b) Could afford up to half a day a month
    (c) Would attend evening sessions occasionally

---

3   What resources are available to support me?

- Is there any money? How much?
- What other resources are available (e.g. people, journals, books)?
- Am I willing/able to contribute to the cost?

  (a) *No money*
  (b) *Might be books at the local library*
  (c) *Could travel to local meetings at my own cost*

---

4   How/where do I learn best?

- What learning experiences have worked really well for me in the past? What made them so successful?
- What learning experiences have I found disappointing? Why?

  (a) *Presentation skills workshop v. good – lots of chance to practise and discuss*
  (b) *PMS conference – talked at all day. Need to ask questions!*

---

5   What will be acceptable at work?

- Am I able to take time-off for a range of personal development activities (e.g. studying at home, visiting another practice, meeting a mentor)?
- Could I undertake my personal development at work (e.g. use the internet at work for e-learning, ask my coach to visit me)?

  (a) *Could take time off to attend relevant meetings*
  (b) *OK to use the internet to search for resources e.g. books etc*

---

6   Who might be able to help me?

- Do you know someone who is an expert in the competence you want to develop?
- Who might know about training and development opportunities in this competence?
- Who else might want to develop this competence?

  (a) *Phil is a great networker – pick his brains?*
  (b) *Jo at Three Firs Surgery – think she attends the local network meeting*
  (c) *Primary care development manager at PCT may be able to help*

Personal development activity 7

Choosing the development methods to meet your needs
Use the *development methods table* and the *developing skills and knowledge matrices* in Section 5 tools to help you identify what you are going to do to meet your training and development needs.

It is important to consider the practical factors and constraints you identified in *personal development activity 6* (*see* p 71) when you are deciding what you are going to do.

Remember to choose a method(s) that:

- takes account of your learning needs, practical resources and any constraints and
- will be effective in helping you develop the competence.

WRITING A PDP

You have now:

- identified the competences that are important in your role now and in the future (*personal development activity 1*, Section 3 – *see* p 30)
- assessed yourself against the competence profile (*personal development activity 2*, Section 4 – *see* p 48)
- gathered information from others about their views of your strengths and development needs against the competence profile (*personal development activity 3*, Section 4 – *see* p 50)
- analysed the information you have gathered and written a list of strengths and development needs (*personal development activity 4*, Section 4 – *see* p 51)
- identified your priority development needs for the next 12 months (*personal development activity 5*, Section 5 – *see* p 70)
- assessed each development need in depth, considering what you need to learn and the practical options open to you (*personal development activity 6*, Section 5 – *see* p 71)
- decided what action you are going to take (*personal development activity 7*, Section 5 – *see* above).

The next step is to put everything into a personal development plan. This will be the tool you use to turn your intentions into action and monitor your progress over the next 12 months.

There are many personal development plan formats and a number of examples are given in Section 5 tools for you to choose from. Select one that meets your requirements, or invent your own. The only criterion is that you use a format that makes sense to you and you can work with.

Personal development activity 8

Writing your personal development plan
Find somewhere quiet where you will not be disturbed and write your plan. Even though you probably have a clear idea in your head at the moment of what you are going to do *it is important that you write everything down* – not only because you are less likely to forget something but because research has shown that we are much more likely to do something if it is written down.

If you have a supportive line manager he or she may be able to help you by offering ideas and practical support. If you want to implement some of your plan during the working day your line manager's agreement is essential.

If your line manager is unable to offer help putting your plan together, consider if anyone else can help – a local training or development specialist, or a colleague.

Next steps for individuals
Go to Section 6 for ideas to help you get support and keep on track when implementing your personal development plan.

LINE MANAGERS AND TRAINERS

TEAM AND ORGANISATIONAL TRAINING AND DEVELOPMENT PLANS

The purpose of team and organisational training and development plans is to identify actions, and allocate resources and responsibility within an agreed time-scale to ensure the right training and development necessary to achieve team or organisational goals.

Plans usually cover a one-year period, and should be reviewed regularly during the 12 months. If the team or organisation has a training and development strategy, the plan will be drawn directly from the strategy.

For example:

Practice objective
- To reduce doctors' workloads over the next two years by introducing general minor illness clinics led by a specialist nurse practitioner.

Supporting element of the training and development strategy
- To develop and run an in-house NVQ training programme for healthcare assistants (HCAs) to support existing practice nurses.

Section of the training and development plan
- Establish arrangements for NVQ assessments for in-house HCA programme. Two practice nurses to become internal assessors and achieve A1 by August 2004. Cost £X.

If the team or organisation does not have longer-term plans and strategies, the training and development plan may be based on:

- annual business plans
- changes or developments planned for the next year, e.g.:
  - new services for patients
  - new management or administrative systems
  - NHS developments affecting the team/practice – National Service Frameworks (NSFs).

Manager's/trainer's activity 7

Developing a team or organisational training plan
1 Use your strategy and/or any other team or organisational plans to identify action to be taken in the next 12 months.
2 Identify the options for meeting the needs and estimate costs.
3 Collate and review personal development plans and identify any training and development needs that are common to a number of staff. Identify options and estimate costs for meeting these needs.

  Note: It may be more effective to organise a training programme to be run in-house, or to buy training materials (e.g. CD-ROM), where a number of staff have listed the same need on their personal development plan. It is important to consider all the practicalities before going ahead – what would the implications for the team/practice be if all staff participated in training at the same time; would staff benefit from undertaking the training with people from other organisations?

If it is not appropriate to buy-in a workshop or materials, co-ordinating personal development plans and identifying common needs will enable you to negotiate discounts where more than one member of staff is attending over the next few months.

4 Calculate the cost of your plan – is it within the available budget? If not, review your plan:

- Are there any activities that could be provided through less expensive options? Could one person attend a course and train others with the same need?
- What are the priorities that must be met? What areas could be deferred until next year?

5 Agree the plan with the team or key stakeholders in the organisation.

See Section 5 tools for a training and development plan template and example plan.

Team development

Developing a team or organisational training and development plan may lead to the identification of a need for general team development or building. This may result from:

- a number of new people joining the team or organisation and the need to 'get to know each other'
- changes that have led or will lead to a need to reassess how everyone in the team or organisation works together – new or expanded premises, or new services, for example
- a general feeling of 'needing to take stock'.

If you have identified a need for general team development it is important to be very clear about what you want to achieve, in order to select the best method and get the outcome(s) you want. See the *identifying objectives for team development checklist* and *team development methods* in Section 5 tools.

Section 5

THE TOOLS

ASSESSING NEEDS AND OPTIONS

Competence:
1   What do I need?
• How much do I already know? Am I starting from scratch? • Do I need to develop my knowledge? • Do I understand the theory but need to practise? • Could I practise on the job, or do I need a low-risk environment away from work?
2   How much time do I have?
• How quickly do I need the competence? Do I need it urgently? • Can I afford to take time away from work to develop it? How much? • Am I prepared to spend some of my own time developing it?
3   What resources are available to support me?
• Is there any money? How much? • What other resources are available (e.g. people, journals, books)? • Am I willing/able to contribute to the cost?

---

4   How/where do I learn best?

- What learning experiences have worked really well for me in the past? What made them so successful?
- What learning experiences have I found disappointing? Why?

---

5   What will be acceptable at work?

- Am I able to take time off for a range of personal development activities (e.g. studying at home, visiting another practice, meeting a mentor)?
- Could I undertake my personal development at work (e.g. use the internet at work for e-learning, ask my coach to visit me)?

---

6   Who might be able to help me?

- Do you know someone who is an expert in the competence you want to develop?
- Who might know about training and development opportunities in this competence?
- Who else might want to develop this competence?

DEVELOPING SKILLS AND KNOWLEDGE MATRICES

The developing skills and knowledge matrices on the following pages suggest some of the methods that can be used to develop the underpinning skills and knowledge of the practice management competence profile.

They will help you choose from the range of options that are available to meet your development needs.

You will find descriptions of all the development methods listed in the matrices and particular points to consider in the *development methods table* on pages 86–89.

DEVELOPING SKILLS MATRIX

	Assertiveness	Chairing meetings	Coaching	Conflict management	Creativity	Decision making	Delegation	Facilitation	Feedback – giving/receiving	Influencing	Interviewing	Listening	Mentoring
Workshops		×				×				×			
Voluntary work		×										×	×
Secondments													
Role model	×					×				×			
Reading			×									×	
Questionnaires	×												
Project work										×	×		
Professional qualifications											×		
Professional/ statutory bodies									×				
Open learning						×	×						
Mentor				×					×				×
Job swap								×					
Evening classes					×								
E-learning			×		×								
Conferences			×				×						×
Co-consultancy				×		×		×	×				
Coaching	×									×			
Audio/video tapes		×			×								
Action learning				×				×				×	

	Motivating others	Negotiation	Networking	Note taking	Numerical	Objective setting	Planning	Prioritisation	Problem solving	Project management	Questioning	Report writing	Stress management	Team building	Time management
Workshops						×					×				
Voluntary work				×				×							
Secondments															
Role model												×		×	
Reading			×						×						×
Questionnaires													×		
Project work				×			×			×					
Professional qualifications		×			×										
Professional/ statutory bodies		×	×					×							
Open learning	×						×			×					
Mentor			×					×						×	
Job swap	×									×		×			
Evening classes				×	×							×	×		
E-learning		×				×					×				
Conferences						×									×
Co-consultancy									×						
Coaching	×				×										×
Audio/video tapes							×						×		
Action learning									×	×				×	

DEVELOPING KNOWLEDGE MATRIX

	Appointments systems	Appraisal processes	Book keeping	Business planning	Change management	Complaints procedures	Data protection regulations	Dealing with aggression	Employment law	Health and safety regulations	Human resources practice	Identifying training needs	Income/expenditure accounts	Items of service (IOS)
Workshops		×						×		×				
Voluntary work														
Secondments														
Role model					×									
Reading				×			×		×				×	×
Questionnaires	×													
Project work												×		
Professional qualifications			×						×					
Professional/statutory bodies						×	×		×	×				
Open learning		×		×							×			
Mentor					×						×			
Job swap	×													
Evening classes			×										×	
E-learning				×								×		
Conferences						×	×					×		
Co-consultancy						×		×		×				×
Coaching	×							×					×	
Audio/video tapes		×	×								×			
Action learning					×									

	Networks local/national	NHS developments	Non-verbal communication	PAYE	Personal medical services	Red book	Rota systems	Self awareness	Statutory maternity pay	Statutory sick pay	Training methods
Workshops											×
Voluntary work											
Secondments											
Role model			×								
Reading		×			×	×					
Questionnaires								×			
Project work							×				
Professional qualifications				×							×
Professional/ statutory bodies	×	×		×					×	×	
Open learning											
Mentor	×							×			
Job swap					×		×				
Evening classes											
E-learning		×									
Conferences			×								
Co-consultancy	×			×							×
Coaching					×	×	×		×	×	
Audio/video tapes			×								
Action learning								×			

DEVELOPMENT METHODS TABLE

This table lists a wide range of development methods that can be used to help develop primary care practice management competences. Use it to help you identify what you will do to meet your training and development needs.

Development method	What it is	Points to consider
Action learning	A group of people – usually six to eight – work together to help one another learn from their work experiences.	Action learning groups or sets usually meet every six to eight weeks over a number of months, or even years. They are useful for helping to learn through work experience. An effective way of developing learning and self-development skills and for gaining insight into group working and facilitation.
Audio/video tapes	Training seminars and workshops on audio and video; some 'speaking books' on audio. Some are supported by workbooks.	A flexible way of learning – videos can be played at work or home and audio tapes can be played in the car. Not interactive so need to be supported by other methods for discussion of ideas or for feedback on development of competence.
Coaching	Coaching is a relationship between two people where someone who is an expert in an area helps the other person to develop his or her competence. Usually a short-term relationship.	A good coach will give guidance on how to develop skills/knowledge, provide encouragement and support and offer feedback to help development. A colleague may provide this service without charging, but professionals will charge a fee. *See* Section 6 for more details.
Co-consultancy	Two colleagues of a similar level work together to provide each other with advice, support and feedback.	Important to have a clear agreement of what your objectives are and ground rules for operating the relationship. *See* Section 6 for more details.

Conferences	Formal events organised to provide information about or explore issues surrounding a topic.	Good way of gaining access to experts although opportunities for questioning and discussion in plenary and workshop sessions will vary. Good for networking and making contacts. Always important to ensure the conference objectives will meet your specific needs.
E-learning	Learning using computer-based technology e.g. CD-ROM, interactive video and internet.	Flexible way of gaining skills and knowledge if you have access to IT resources. Some local libraries offer access to hardware and software. Degree of interaction varies, but many provide at least limited feedback to learners.
Evening/weekend classes	Formal courses organised by schools, colleges and universities during evenings and weekends. Can last from one session upwards, and may lead to the award of qualifications.	Good option if time off from work for training and development activities is difficult.
Job swaps	Two people of a similar level in different jobs exchange roles for a period of time to gain experience and develop new competences.	Way to gain new experiences and competences on the job. Can advertise in local newsletters for a job swap partner if there is no obvious candidate.
Mentor	A mentor helps another person develop by sharing his or her experience and expertise. Usually a long-term relationship.	Mentoring is used to describe a variety of approaches and it is vital to be clear about what is needed. *See* Section 6 for more details.
Open, distance and flexible learning	Ways of learning that are flexible to individual needs (e.g. the time, place, style of learning and length of time of the course). May lead to the award of qualifications.	Very flexible way of gaining competences – allow for study at home or at work; some programmes offered by educational institutions will have set timetables. Availability of feedback varies – but may be face to face, by correspondence or via internet.

Development method	What it is	Points to consider
Professional bodies	Institutions and associations that represent a particular profession. Generally offer a wide range of services to members and some for non-members.	Some institutions offer short courses and seminars in their specialist area, e.g. Chartered Institute of Personnel and Development, Institute of Health Management.
Professional qualifications	Formal courses of study leading to the award of qualifications and/or membership of the professional body.	Courses of study offered by human resources, accountancy and health management bodies are relevant to primary care practice management and will open other career development options.
Project work and working group membership	Taking on a project or specific responsibilities as a member of a working group for a period of time to gain new experience and develop competence.	Activities usually undertaken in addition to current role, therefore need to consider workload implications carefully. Need to be clear about deadlines and expectations. Good for making contacts and networking as well as gaining experience and new competence.
Questionnaires	Personality and ability questionnaires can provide a way of gaining feedback on the development of competence and signpost further development needs.	Can be a helpful way of gaining insight and self-awareness.
Reading	Learning from books, journals, internet etc.	Flexible, often relatively cheap, gives access to a wide range of ideas and opinions. Some local libraries offer a range of management and personal development texts. Need to supplement with other methods for discussion of ideas and feedback on development.

Role model	Consciously observing and emulating the behaviour of an individual who displays excellence in a competence or range of competences.	May simply observe the role model's behaviour and adopt it (e.g. watching an expert chairperson in action at a meeting, analysing what he or she does and adopting the behaviour) or may seek a more formal arrangement – e.g. spend a day with him or her, ask for coaching.
Secondment	Taking on a different job in the same or a different organisation for a set period of time (at least weeks and usually months) to gain new experience and develop competences.	Essential to be explicit about needs of both parties and to have clear objectives for the secondment. Important to have good 'keep-in-touch' arrangements with substantive job, including arrangements for returning at the end of the secondment.
Voluntary work or service	Gaining experience or competence through unpaid volunteering.	Good way of gaining competence and experience combined with personal interests. Many opportunities exist for volunteering – e.g. charity fundraising, school governors and PTA, volunteer mentoring and listening schemes.
Workshops, short courses and seminars	Short courses (generally one to five days) aimed at developing competences.	Helpful for acquiring knowledge and skills, and good for practising new skills in a 'safe' environment – although artificiality of situation can hinder. Important to have specific objectives for attending and ensure they will be met by the course curriculum.

PRIMARY CARE MANAGEMENT PROGRAMME MODULES SUPPORTING THE DEVELOPMENT OF PRIMARY CARE PRACTICE MANAGEMENT COMPETENCES

Modules from the Primary Care Management Programme (available from education@radcliffemed.com or tel: 01235 528820) provide resources for developing all primary care practice management competences. This table shows which modules link to each competence area.

Managing work	Working with other people
• Preparing a business plan • Problem and decision analysis • Achieving results through meetings • Effective time management • Health, safety, contract and environmental law • Operations management • Managing patient care • Project management • Managing quality • Resource and facilities management	• Negotiating effectively • Managing aggression, abuse and violence
Managing change	**Communicating**
• Managing change	• Communicating effectively • Appraising and counselling staff • Managing marketing and public relations
Managing other people	**Analysing and using data**
• Leading a team • Employment law • Appraising and counselling staff • Recruiting and selecting people • Disciplinary and grievance procedures	• Remuneration planning • Financial planning • Financial performance and control • Understanding financial statements • Information management
Developing other people	**Personal effectiveness**
• Training and developing people	• Training and developing people

PERSONAL DEVELOPMENT PLAN FORMAT 1

What I need to learn . . .

Why I need to learn it . . .

How I am going to learn it . . .

I will start . . .

I will finish . . .

I will get help from . . .

PERSONAL DEVELOPMENT PLAN FORMAT 2

1 Managing work: objective		
Action to be taken:	Start date:	End date:
2 Managing change: objective		
Action to be taken:	Start date:	End date:
3 Managing other people: objective		
Action to be taken:	Start date:	End date:
4 Developing other people: objective		
Action to be taken:	Start date:	End date:

5 Working with other people: objective		
Action to be taken:	Start date:	
	End date:	
6 Communicating: objective		
Action to be taken:	Start date:	
	End date:	
7 Analysing and using data: objective		
Action to be taken:	Start date:	
	End date:	
8 Personal effectiveness: objective		
Action to be taken:	Start date:	
	End date:	

PERSONAL DEVELOPMENT PLAN FORMAT 3

Learning objective	Method(s) to meet objective	Action	Resources	Review date	Achieve by

PERSONAL DEVELOPMENT PLAN FORMAT 4

Personal development plan

My objective is . . . .

. . . .

. . . .

What I am going to do
(List all action steps)

. . . .

. . . .

. . . .

. . . .

. . . .

My next steps:
Tomorrow I will . . . .
Over the next week I will . . . .

. . . .

. . . .

Over the next month I will . . . .

. . . .

. . . .

Over the next three months I will . . . .

. . . .

. . . .

. . . .

I will achieve my objective by . . . . (Date)

TEAM OR ORGANISATIONAL TRAINING AND DEVELOPMENT PLAN TEMPLATE

Objective	Action	Timescale	Resources	Action by

EXAMPLE PRACTICE TRAINING AND DEVELOPMENT PLAN

Objective	Action	Timescale	Resources	Action by
To ensure all new staff receive comprehensive induction to the practice and their job	• Develop new general induction pack for all new staff • Review arrangements for locum GPs	By 30.6.0X By 30.9.0X	N/A	Practice Manager Practice Manager and Senior Partner
Promote zero tolerance approach and ensure all practice staff know how to handle violence or abuse from patients	• Four staff to attend workshop organised by local PCT	By 31.12.0X	£X00	Head Receptionist
Support the development of nurse practitioner-led general minor illness clinics	• Healthcare assistants to achieve level 3 in Direct Care NVQ	By 31.3.0X	£X00	Senior Nurse Practitioner
Ensure all clinical staff are aware of diabetes NSF and implications for the practice	• Awareness raising session at monthly meeting	By 30.4.0X	N/A	Dr Jones

IDENTIFYING OBJECTIVES FOR TEAM DEVELOPMENT CHECKLIST

PURPOSE

Use this checklist to identify specific objectives for team building or development activities. This will enable you to select the most appropriate method(s) to meet your team's needs.

	Purpose of team development	*Yes/No*
1	For all team members to learn new skills and/or knowledge? Note: Do all members of the team need the same level of skill/knowledge? If not, could some people feel bored or intimidated by some of the activity? Is a whole team event the best way of achieving the objective?	
2	To make decisions about the future direction of the team? Note: Is it clear who has the power to make decisions and who does not?	
3	To generate ideas and plans for the future?	
4	To make everyone feel involved and part of the team?	
5	To improve relationships within the team?	
6	To work out solutions to operational problems?	
7	To consult team members about a proposal or plan?	
8	Other – insert details:	

TEAM DEVELOPMENT METHODS

Method	Description	Points to consider
'Awaydays' or 'timeouts'	The whole team/all members of the organisation spend a substantial period of time (a day or 24-hour period) together, away from the workplace, to work together on an issue of shared interest and concern and/or to build/develop team relationships. Awaydays are often used to develop goals, objectives and plans, and/or build/develop working relationships. A facilitator who is skilled in group processes and not a member of the team may be used to help ensure the event achieves its goals.	Awaydays are an effective way of increasing involvement and ownership of team objectives where the agenda and process means everyone has the opportunity and capability to contribute. Junior members of a team may feel disengaged from the process if they spend the majority of their time listening to the discussions of senior staff. Careful consideration should be given to who should facilitate the process, particularly if the agenda will be exploring roles, responsibilities and relationships in the team. A good external facilitator will have the skills and experience to deal with any conflicts that arise. He/she is also more likely to be viewed as impartial by all team members.
Social events	Any voluntary social occasion attended by team members (with or without partners).	Social events can be an effective way of developing relationships in the team, allowing members to get to know one another outside the context of work roles. Participation should always be voluntary.

Method	Description	Points to consider
Team building events	Activities, often outdoors, that give all participants the opportunity to work together as a team to achieve an objective or engage in an unfamiliar activity. Some (e.g. outward-bound) focus on giving participants experience of leadership (and followership); others are intended simply as an enjoyable shared experience, e.g. go-carting, paintballing.	Can provide a good way of building relationships as team members see each other in a different context and new roles. It is important to choose an activity that all team members have the physical capability to participate in. Participation should always be voluntary – even if in normal working hours.
Joint learning	This may include the team participating in a course or workshop together, or making a visit to another team/practice to learn about their good practices.	Team development is generally a useful by-product of joint learning events rather than the purpose for organising them since all participants should genuinely have a need for the training and development. Visits can be a particularly useful way for team members to fulfil differing needs at the same time (i.e. learning about the aspects of another organisation's good practice that are relevant to them).
Projects	Members of a team work together for a period of time on a specific project.	Team development is generally a useful by-product of the project rather than its purpose. Joint working on a project can lead to increased understanding and appreciation of skills and experience. It is important that all participants have shared objectives and are clear about their own roles and responsibilities.

Team meetings	Regular, planned meetings where all members of the team contribute to decision making, problem solving and share information about their current activities.	The purpose of team meetings should be agreed and reviewed regularly. A wish to include everyone needs to be balanced against the contribution individuals are able to make. Some members may attend for only part of the meeting.
Psychometric or personality questionnaires	Questionnaires that provide insights into individual preferences and styles of working – for example, Myers Briggs Type Instrument (MBTI), Belbin Team Roles.	Can help develop relationships by increasing understanding of the preferences of team members. Some questionnaires can only be administered/interpreted after training.

Section 6

IMPLEMENTING DEVELOPMENT PLANS

PURPOSE

This section gives practical suggestions for implementing individual, team and organisational development plans and tackling blocks and problems if they arise.

PERSONAL DEVELOPMENT

PERSONAL DEVELOPMENT PLANNING

Preparing a good personal development plan can be very hard work, but successful implementation can be even harder. It is not at all unusual for really good plans to remain just that and never get turned into action. Taking action in three key areas will help make sure you achieve your objectives:

- finding the people who can and will help you
- getting the most from development activities
- reviewing progress regularly (*see* Section 7).

Finding the people who can and will help you
You may need the help of others in a number of ways:

- for encouragement
- for advice, guidance and ideas
- to open doors, and make contacts
- to review progress and develop your plan

- to provide resources
- for information about opportunities locally.

Other people may fulfil a number of helpful roles:

- line manager
- mentor
- coach
- co-consultant.

Line managers

A supportive line manager is an invaluable asset. Some are very skilled at helping others develop; however, many line managers want to help but are not sure how to go about it. This can sometimes result in a manager appearing unsupportive when he or she simply lacks the skills, knowledge or confidence to offer help.

Personal development activity 9

Helping your line manager help you
Think about how you might use the resources in this tool kit to help your line manager help you – for example, clarifying your current role and how it might change by working through the *competence profile* together (Section 3 tools), providing feedback using the *competence assessment questionnaire* (Section 4 tools), discussing possible development options using the *developing skills and knowledge matrices* or the *development methods table* (Section 5 tools).

However, some managers do not have either the skills or the motivation to develop their staff and in these circumstances gaining support from others becomes vital – although additional external help can be essential even with a supportive boss.

Mentors

WHAT IS MENTORING?

Mentoring is a term used to describe a variety of different approaches, but at its core is a relationship between two people, one of whom has the explicit role of helping the other person develop by sharing his or her experience and expertise. It is usually a long-term relationship, lasting months and even years.

HOW CAN A MENTOR HELP?

A mentor may help by:

- providing personal support and guidance
- giving training, development and career advice
- helping with networking and making introductions
- supporting problem solving, challenging thinking and encouraging new ideas.

A mentor may be able to provide effective help in all these areas while others may only be able or willing to help in some.

SUCCESSFUL MENTORING

To find the right mentor for you and then work together:

- be clear about why you want a mentor and what you need from one
- ensure your mentor understands your expectations and you understand the mentor's
- agree and stick to ground rules for how you will work together.

HOW TO FIND A MENTOR

It can be helpful to think about 'recruiting' a mentor in the same way as you would a new member of staff.

1   Use the *identifying a mentor checklist* in Section 6 tools to help you think through what you want your mentor to do and jot down a 'job description' for the mentor.
2   Develop a person specification for your ideal mentor – decide what is essential to you and what is only desirable. This will help you clarify the type of person you should be looking for or may help you assess someone you already have in mind before you approach them. It may be helpful to consider the following questions:
    - Do I have a preference about my mentor's gender? Could I work with a man or a woman?
    - What experience will he/she need (e.g. working in primary care, a senior management role, a general management role, human resources, finance etc.)?
    - Does my mentor need to have a good up-to-date understanding of primary care? The wider NHS?
3   Consider any practical issues. For example:
    - How far am I prepared to travel to see my mentor? (It is usual for the mentee to travel to see his/her mentor.)
4   If you already have someone in mind as a possible mentor, measure what you know about him or her against your 'job description' and 'person specification'. If he or she looks like a good match, contact the person to ask

if he or she would be willing to meet you to discuss becoming your mentor. Having an initial 'no commitments' meeting is important to avoid difficulties and embarrassment if you and your mentor are not a good 'match'.

If the person says no, or you don't have any ideas about possible mentors, you may be able to identify someone by:

- asking contacts in other practices or your PCT if they can suggest someone
- tapping into a mentor scheme run by healthcare organisations locally – contact the human resources department at the nearest hospital trust or shared services agency. Even if they don't run a formal scheme, some human resources departments may be willing to suggest contacts.

This meeting gives you a chance to get to know each other, and to decide if you can work together. It is the time to clarify what you both want from the relationship and agree future ground rules. Use the *developing a mentoring agreement* checklist in Section 6 tools to help you do this.

5   Once you have agreed to go ahead, write up your agreement and send a copy to your mentor to check that you have the same understanding of what will happen.

This may sound too formal (and in some situations it could be, so you need to use your judgement) but it does avoid any danger of misunderstanding later on.

Coaching

WHAT IS COACHING?

Coaching is a relationship between two people, where someone with a high level of expertise in a specific area helps another person develop his or her competence. It is usually a short-term relationship, which ends when the competence is developed. We are familiar with the concept from sports, but it is increasingly used in business as a formal tool for management and personal development.

Professional coaches charge for their services, but it is also possible to get effective coaching from colleagues who may see giving such help to others as part of their job and not ask for payment.

Coaching is different from mentoring, which is usually a longer-term relationship with a wider focus, but part of what a mentor does may be coaching.

HOW CAN A COACH HELP?

A coach may help by:

- providing expert advice and guidance on how to develop a specific competence

- giving encouragement and support
- offering feedback on performance.

Coaching may be helpful in a number of ways:

- if you are faced with a new situation where advice and guidance from an expert will help you 'learn as you go' and ensure success (for example, handling a discipline or grievance for the first time)
- developing a new competence (for example, developing a team)
- improving performance in a particular area (for example, chairing meetings, preparing for interviews).

SUCCESSFUL COACHING

To find the right coach for you and then work successfully with him or her you must:

- be clear about what you need from a coach
- ensure your coach understands your expectations and you understand the coach's
- agree and stick to ground rules for how you will work together.

HOW TO FIND A COACH

Use the *finding a coach checklist* in Section 5 tools to help you identify and recruit a coach.

Co-consultancy

WHAT IS CO-CONSULTANCY?

Co-consultancy is where two people of the same or similar levels have a formal agreement to work together to provide each other with help with personal development and problem solving. The partners meet regularly to discuss experiences, share ideas and give each other feedback.

A co-consultancy relationship is different from that with a line manager, coach or mentor because of the equal investment made by both parties, who are both entering the relationship to give and receive support, advice and feedback.

The arrangement has many similarities to friendship and sometimes friends will provide each other with informal co-consultancy but it is important to remember it is a different relationship. Co-consultancy will not necessarily develop or support an existing friendship and it may be better to work with a respected, objective colleague with whom you do not have the added ties of friendship.

SUCCESSFUL CO-CONSULTANCY

The foundations of successful co-consultancy are:

- explicit, shared and agreed objectives between both partners, which are openly monitored and regularly reviewed
- mutual trust, respect and honesty
- shared understanding of the ground rules – what is within and without the boundaries of the relationship
- genuine commitment to invest in the relationship – giving and receiving.

Working with someone else in co-consultancy can be a particularly effective way of supporting the implementation of a personal development plan over a number of months or even years.

Personal development activity 10

Identifying who can and will help you implement your personal development plan

Think about the help you need to implement your PDP and who may be able to give it. It can be useful to think in terms of:

- *who knows* about the competence you want to develop, or about opportunities that may be helpful to you
- *who cares* about you and/or your development
- *who will be motivated* enough to give you their time and help.

Make a list of the people you are going to ask for help and what you need from them. Unless you are very lucky it is unlikely that everyone you ask will be able to help so it is a good idea to try to think of more than one person in each area.

Getting the most from development activities
Whatever method(s) you have chosen to meet your training and development need(s) you must be sure that you are clear about what your expectations are and what else is needed to make sure that you can apply what you learn to your job.

You might also want to think about how other people in your practice – your staff or other colleagues – might benefit from what you have learnt.

Before you begin a planned training or development activity (for example, attending a workshop or conference) ask yourself five questions:

- Why is this activity important for my development?
- What will I do differently at work as a result?
- What information shall I share with others in the practice and how might it be used?
- Who can help me use my new skills/knowledge when I return to work?
- How and when will I know if the activity meets my objectives?

This will help you identify any action you need to take *before* and *after* the development activity to help make sure it is a worthwhile investment of your time and effort.

You will also find it helpful to identify the answers to these questions before approaching your line manager or anyone else you are seeking sponsorship from for training and development activities.

LINE MANAGERS AND TRAINERS

TEAM AND ORGANISATIONAL TRAINING AND DEVELOPMENT PLANS: INTERNAL OR EXTERNAL PROVIDERS?

The decision about which parts of the plan can be designed and run by members of the team or organisation and which, if any, by someone from outside (a training consultant or someone from another organisation) is the first step in implementation.

The following factors should be considered when making a decision.

- Are the skills/knowledge/experience to provide the development available internally?
- What are the costs of a member of staff providing the development – e.g. his or her time; what will be the impact on his or her workload and/or that of colleagues?

- Are there any benefits of a member of staff providing the development – e.g. experience, development for him or her?
- Are there any barriers to the development being provided by a member of the team – e.g. credibility, lack of independence?
- What resources will be needed to bring in help from outside the team/ organisation, e.g. time to find and select an external expert, finance if using an external consultant.
- Are the skills/knowledge/experience available outside the team/organisation?
- What are the potential benefits and drawbacks of using external help – e.g. credibility as an expert, independence, a fresh approach, lack of understanding of the context/issues?
- What might the consequences be of an external provider failing to deliver?

External training and development providers

The process that led to the decision to use an external provider of training and development will have clarified the reason that outside help is to be used.

- They add to the internal capacity – an extra pair of hands. You have the necessary technical expertise in-house, but not the time to design and/or run the training.
- They have skills, knowledge and experience that is not held internally.
- They will bring independence and a 'fresh pair of eyes'.

Whatever your reason(s) for deciding to seek external help, it is vital that you specify precisely what you want before entering into an agreement, whether or not you will be paying for the person's services.

The specification should describe:

- the training and development need
- the outcomes to be achieved
- how they are to be achieved
- the boundaries of the assignment.

You may want to leave scope for the person providing the training and development to make proposals about how the outcomes are to be achieved. In this case it is even more important to be very precise about the other three points to avoid any danger of ending up with what someone else wants to provide, rather than what the team or organisation needs.

A *training and development specification framework* and *tender analysis framework* are given in Section 6 tools.

Section 6

THE TOOLS

IDENTIFYING A MENTOR CHECKLIST

Use this checklist to help you identify what you want from a mentor.

Consider the following list of 20 ways a mentor might help and put a tick against the ones that are *most* important for you.

☐ Acts as a sounding board for my ideas

☐ Challenges and questions me

☐ Helps me deal with challenges at work by pushing me to think things through

☐ Advises me on professional issues

☐ Advises me on personal issues relating to my development

☐ Advises me about my training and development needs

☐ Offers me constructive feedback

☐ Will help me solve problems and make decisions

☐ Provides information about developments in primary care

☐ Provides information about developments in the wider NHS

☐ Gives me advice on how to network and make contacts

☐ Encourages me when things are tough

☐ Pushes me to think differently about problems and opportunities

☐ Challenges my assumptions about people and things

☐ Acts as a role model for me

☐ Helps me understand my job in the wider context

☐ Provides career development advice

☐ Introduces me to other people who might help me

☐ Is available to advise me in a personal crisis

☐ Can help me decide how to tackle problems with my staff

Review the items you have ticked. Do they point to a particular type of support you need from a mentor?

DEVELOPING A MENTORING AGREEMENT CHECKLIST

☐ What is the purpose of the relationship?

☐ What does the mentee need?

☐ What can the mentor offer?

☐ What are the mentor's expectations?

☐ What are our objectives?

☐ Are there any areas that we have agreed fall outside the boundaries of our relationship?

☐ What are our rules on confidentiality?

☐ What are our responsibilities (e.g. commitment not to cancel meetings)?

☐ How long will we work together? (Set an end date even if you subsequently decide to extend it.)

☐ When will we review how well things are working?

☐ Where will we meet?

☐ Who is responsible for arranging meetings?

☐ How long will meetings last?

FINDING A COACH CHECKLIST

1   Make a list of what you want from coaching

☐ What are your goals?

☐ What sort of issues will you want to discuss with your coach?

☐ What feedback do you want or need?

☐ What issues of confidentiality might arise?

☐ What resources do you have – time, money, ability to travel?

2   Identify possible coaches

☐ What about people you already know – is one of them an expert in the area you want to develop? – Would he or she coach you?

☐ Who might know of someone who could help you?

☐ Could a professional association or institution offer advice?

3   Approach your potential coach and ask if he or she can help – be very clear about:

☐ What you are trying to achieve.

☐ Why you are approaching him or her.

☐ How you would want to work with the coach.

☐ If the coach will charge for his or her services and how much.

4   If the coach says 'yes', agree the ground rules

☐ Frequency, length and venue for meetings.

☐ Can you contact the coach by e-mail, telephone?

☐ How you will handle confidentiality.

SOURCES OF HELP

There are many sources of help you can tap into for support and ideas. Here are a few suggestions to give you a start.

PROFESSIONAL BODIES AND ASSOCIATIONS

Human Resources
- **The Chartered Institute of Personnel and Development (CIPD)**
  Professional body for human resource and training professionals.
  www.cipd.co.uk
  Tel: 020 8971 9000

Accountancy and Financial Management
- **Association of Chartered Certified Accountants (ACCA)**
  www.acca.org.uk
  Tel: 020 7396 5800
- **Chartered Institute of Management Accountants (CIMA)**
  www.cima.org.uk
  Tel: 020 7663 5441
- **Chartered Institute of Public Finance and Accountancy (CIPFA)**
  www.cipfa.org.uk
  Tel: 020 7543 5600
- **Association of Accounting Technicians (AAT)**
  Trains, supports and develops accounting technicians who work alongside chartered accountants (e.g. as accounts clerks, financial managers). Awards National Vocational Qualifications (NVQs) in accounting.
  www.aat.co.uk
  Tel: 020 7837 8600

Healthcare Associations
- **Healthcare Financial Management Association (HFMA)**
  Organisation for financial healthcare professionals (qualified and unqualified). Members predominantly from the NHS.
  www.hfma.org.uk
  Tel: 0117 929 4789
- **Association of Healthcare Human Resource Management (AHHRM)**
  Aims to bring together healthcare professionals in a nationwide network to

enable them to develop, influence and promote high-quality human resource management in the NHS.
www.ahhrm.org.uk
Tel: 01275 394438

- **Institute of Healthcare Management (IHM)**
  Largest UK professional body for managers working in healthcare and health services. Specialist primary care sub-group of institute 'primary care sector'.
  www.ihm.org.uk
  Tel: 020 7881 9235

USEFUL WEBSITES

This list represents a tiny selection of the websites that may be of help.

Open, distance, flexible and e-learning
- www.open.ac.uk – The Open University.
- www.nec.ac.uk – The National Extension College.
- www.bbc.co.uk/education/home – BBC website.
- www.videoarts.com – Video Arts.

General advice and information
- www.learndirect.co.uk – Government-sponsored initiative supporting online learning; also offers advice line (Tel: 0800 100 900) and national course database.
- www.support4learning.org.uk – website offering learning advice and information.
- www.do-it.org.uk – volunteering website.

Creativity
- www.brainstorming.co.uk – has links to a large number of other sites on brainstorming, creative thinking and innovation.

OTHER IDEAS . . .

- Visit your local library – many have excellent management and business sections and may loan videos, tapes and CD-ROMs as well as books.
- Contact your local volunteer centre – if you don't know where it is, look in the Yellow Pages.
- Contact local schools, colleges, or universities to find out what they can offer.

TRAINING AND DEVELOPMENT SPECIFICATION FRAMEWORK

Inputs	
1	Who is the client (e.g. Practice Manager, PCT)?
2	Who are the users (e.g. all team members)?
3	What resources are available – e.g. money, venue(s) for training etc.?
4	What time is available?
5	List skills, knowledge, experience and values needed by the provider.
6	Background – how was the need identified (e.g. due to planned changes, result of new equipment or services)?
Processes	
1	Identify the roles and tasks of the client, users and provider – e.g. who organises venue?
2	How will communications between the client, users and provider be handled – e.g. will the provider make arrangements direct with users?

3	How will payment be made and when? What expenses will be paid?
4	Any penalty clauses – e.g. for cancellation, failure to deliver materials on time?
5	How will the provider be selected – e.g. written proposal, formal presentation and/or interview, references?

Outcomes

1	What outcomes are required?
2	When will the outcomes be achieved?
3	How will the outcomes be measured, by whom and when – e.g. evaluation process?

Information requested from potential provider(s)

1 Name(s) and CV(s) of staff who will undertake the work.
2 Details of previous relevant experience.
3 Two referees.
4 How they propose to achieve the outcomes.
5 Breakdown of costs.
6 Their terms of business – e.g. what is their policy on cancellation by you?

TENDER ANALYSIS FRAMEWORK

	Proposal 1	Proposal 2	Proposal 3
Level of skills and knowledge			
Experience – recent, relevant, credible?			
Capacity to deliver the assignment			
Value for money			
How well does proposal meet the specification?			
Added value, e.g. ideas, experience that add to planned outcomes			

Section 7

EVALUATION AND REVIEW

PURPOSE

This section provides guidance and tools on evaluation and review of individual and team training and development.

PERSONAL DEVELOPMENT

REVIEWING PROGRESS AND KEEPING ON TRACK

A personal development plan should be kept under continuous review to monitor progress and spot the need for any changes or additions.

It is a good idea to review your plan at least once a month and have a more in-depth re-evaluation at least once every six months.

- If you have been getting help with the whole plan or part of it from someone else (e.g. line manager, mentor or coach), involve them in your review.
- It can also be helpful to complete the competence assessment questionnaire again, either as a self-assessment or by asking those who gave you feedback before to do so again. You can then compare the two sets of feedback and review your progress.

Be as objective as you can when reviewing your successes and any setbacks. A review format is provided in Section 7 tools.

LINE MANAGERS AND TRAINERS

EVALUATING INDIVIDUAL, TEAM AND ORGANISATIONAL TRAINING AND DEVELOPMENT

Purpose
The purpose of evaluating training and development activities is to inform future action, not to review the past. Effective evaluation will make sure that you continue doing what works and abandon that which does not.

Deciding what to evaluate
The first step in a worthwhile evaluation of training and development activities is to decide what you want to know and why – that is:

1 Impact
  - Reactions to the training – did the trainee(s) enjoy the training and think it was valid and that it met their needs?
  - Learning from the training – did the trainee(s) learn what they needed to?
  - Changes in performance – has the learning been applied on the job?
  - Impact on objectives – have the job or business objectives that led to the training need been met?
2 Cost
  - How much did it cost to achieve the objective? Consider total costs – trainees' time (salary costs), trainer's/speaker's fees, cost of venue, refreshments, materials etc.
  - Was the objective achieved in an efficient way? Costs of other options?
  - Were the costs worth the benefits? Did the impact of the training make the investment of total costs worthwhile?

It may not be realistic to measure costs and benefits down to the last penny, but even forming a fairly rough estimate will help to determine whether the training or development was worthwhile and provide lessons for the future.

Evaluation methods
The choice of evaluation method will depend on what is to be evaluated and why. A number of methods and suggested applications are provided in Section 7 tools.

Evaluating training plans
In addition to reviewing each objective of the training plan it may be useful to develop an overview of the cost and benefits of the whole plan. This can be done using the 'Boston Square' technique.

For example:

Impact		
High		
	PCT zero tolerance workshop	Practice awayday In-house NVQ programme
	Awareness-raising session on diabetes NSF New induction arrangements for locum GPs	New induction pack
Low		
	Low	**High**
	Cost	

This allows you to identify common themes between those activities that resulted in a high or low impact.

Section 7
THE TOOLS

Reviewing progress and next steps

- What was my original objective?

- What did I do to meet it?

- What happened?

- Why did it happen?

- What am I going to do now?

EVALUATION METHODS AND USES

Method	Description	Suggestions for use
Post-course questionnaires	Questionnaires given to participants to complete immediately at the end of a course or workshop, asking for their views on the training.	Useful for measuring reactions to training – provide immediate, structured feedback. Can be particularly useful when using a new provider for the first time, or for training that is due to be repeated. Quick, easy method. Usually get a high return rate if participants are asked to complete before leaving. Not useful for measuring learning or application.
Follow-up questionnaires	Questionnaires given/sent to participants some time (week, month, six months) after training, seeking information on what they learnt and how it has been applied to their job. May also be sent to participants' line managers.	Useful for measuring learning and application to job role. Sending to line managers may provide evaluation of changes to job performance and contribution to objectives. Return rate may not be high – provision of a stamped addressed envelope sometimes helps.
Interview	Telephone or face-to-face interview with trainees after completion of training. May be carried out more than once, i.e. immediately after, one month and six months. May also interview line managers.	Useful for assessing all types of impact from reactions to objectives depending on when carried out. Allows flexibility to follow up particular issues. Taking the initiative to arrange the interview generally gives a high participation rate. Can be time consuming.

Method	Description	Suggestions for use
Observation	Observing the individual apply the new skills or knowledge.	Useful if accurate application of new skills is critical, e.g. inputting data, or to provide feedback and suggestions for further development, e.g. presentation skills. Can be carried out by the line manager or an appropriately skilled colleague.
Tests/ simulations	A written or verbal exercise that requires the trainee to apply the new skills/knowledge of the job.	Useful if correct application of new skills/knowledge is critical and observation is inappropriate or not possible, e.g. counselling skills.

INDEX OF ACTIVITIES

INDEX OF TOOLS AND THEIR USES

INDEX